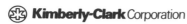

Kimberly-Clark Corporation

Dear Health Care Worker:

Kimberly-Clark Corporation Professional Health Care is pleased to be able to offer you a copy of "Infection Control for the Health Care Worker" by L. G. Donowitz, M.D. This handbook is designed to assist you in your understanding and treatment of diseases that you may encounter in your training and profession.

We hope this book is helpful to you and serves as an important reference for you in your program.

Sincerely,

John S. Metz
President
Professional Health Care
Kimberly-Clark Corporation

For information on KIMBERLY-CLARK™ Personal Protective Equipment, call 1-800-KC-HELPS (1-800-524-3577).

Infection Control
for the
Health Care
Worker

Leigh G. Donowitz

The Children's Medical Center
Professor of Pediatrics
University of Virginia School of Medicine
Charlottesville, Virginia

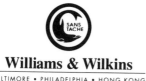

Williams & Wilkins

BALTIMORE • PHILADELPHIA • HONG KONG
LONDON • MUNICH • SYDNEY • TOKYO

A WAVERLY COMPANY

Editor: Jonathan Pine
Managing Editor: Molly L. Mullen
Copy Editor: Shelley Potler
Designer: Wilma Rosenberger
Production Coordinator: Barbara J. Felton
Cover Designer: Wilma Rosenberger

Copyright © 1994
Williams & Wilkins
428 East Preston Street
Baltimore, Maryland 21202, USA

Accurate indications, adverse reactions, and dosage schedules for drugs are provided in this book, but it is possible that they may change. The reader is urged to review the package information data of the manufacturers of the medications mentioned.

Printed in the United States of America

Library of Congress Cataloging-in-Publication Data

Donowitz, Leigh G.
    Infection control for the health care worker / Leigh G. Donowitz.
        p.   cm.
    Includes index.
    ISBN 0-683-02608-9
    1. Nosocomial infections—Prevention—Handbooks, manuals, etc. 2. Medical personnel—Health and hygiene—Handbooks, manuals, etc. I. Title.
    [DNLM: 1. Infection Control—methods—handbooks. 2. Universal Precautions—methods—handbooks. 3. Occupational Health—handbooks. WC 39 D6871 1993]
RA969.D66 1993
614.4'4—dc20   CIP
DNLM/DLC   93–27555
for Library of Congress   93 94 95 96 97
                           1 2 3 4 5 6 7 8 9 10

Dedicated

to Jerry Donowitz

My best friend and foundation

and the finest bedside doctor and teacher I know

PREFACE

There are over 5.5 million health care workers in the United States. All of these workers are exposed to bacteria, viruses, and other infectious agents that can cause mild, severe, and life-threatening infections. Approximately 7500 health care workers are infected with the Hepatitis B virus each year and 300 die of the complications of this infection. The Acquired Immune Deficiency Syndrome (AIDS) epidemic has forced us to carefully evaluate the risks of acquiring the Human Immunodeficiency Virus (HIV) and other high-risk pathogens in the workplace and, most importantly, find methods for preventing such infection.

This guide has been written with the goal of providing each health care worker with a user-friendly, ready reference on the infections that are present in the workplace, how they are transmitted, and the effective infection control methods for preventing such transmission.

It is my sincere wish that this guide makes each health care worker better informed and thus better prepared to knowledgeably, comfortably, and safely care for all patients.

Leigh G. Donowitz, M.D.

CONTENTS

chapter 1

HOW PATHOGENS ARE SPREAD

Outpatient and inpatient health care facilities provide a unique setting that is conducive to transmission of infectious agents. Easy and practical methods to prevent transmission of pathogens in the health care workplace are available but this requires an understanding of how transmission occurs.

Three steps are required for transmission of an infectious agent from an infected individual to an uninfected person (Table 1.1). First, the pathogen must be excreted by the infected person from a site such as the nose, the mouth, or in the feces. Second, the excreted pathogen must be transferred across to the well person. Transfer could be through the air (aerosol spread), by direct contact (hand holding), or by way of an intermediary surface (door knobs). Finally, the infecting agent must reach a susceptible site (usually the mouth, the nose, or the eye) in order to infect the well person. A pathogen on the skin of a well person does not infect that person unless it is inoculated on to a susceptible skin or mucosal surface.

The sites from which organisms are excreted by an infected patient are known. **DIRECT** transfer of pathogens occurs when infected or infested skin (e.g., impetigo, varicella,

Table 1.1.
Three Steps Required for Transmission of Infectious Agent[a]
from Infected Patient to Uninfected Health Care Worker

Excretion	Pathogen must be excreted from site(s) by infected patient
Transfer	Pathogen must be transferred to health care worker
Inoculation	Pathogen must reach susceptible site in the health care worker

[a]Infectious agent = bacteria, viruses, parasites.

lice) is in direct contact or via fomite spread with susceptible skin of the health care worker. **RESPIRATORY** transmission of viruses and bacteria are excreted in respiratory tract secretions (nasal mucus, droplets in cough or sneezes). **FECAL-ORAL** transmission of pathogens, which infect the gastrointestinal tract, are usually excreted in the feces. **BLOODBORNE** pathogens, such as Hepatitis B and human immunodeficiency virus (HIV), are in blood and blood-containing body fluids and are spread by blood or blood-containing fluid spray onto mucous membranes, inoculated by needlestick or sharp injury, or contamination of a nonintact skin surface. Examples of common hospital pathogens and their mode of transmission to health care personnel are outlined in Table 1.2.

The three transmission steps may be illustrated with two examples. In the first, transmission of a virus causing gastroenteritis (e.g., rotavirus) would begin with excretion of the virus in the diarrheal stool of a sick child. Transfer of the virus to a well health care worker would involve contamination of the person's hands with stool during examination or while changing the diaper of the infant. The final step, inoculation of a susceptible site, requires that the health care worker put his or her hands or contaminated articles into the mouth. The virus then would infect the lower gastrointesti-

Table 1.2.
Examples of Common Hospital Pathogens and Mode of Transmission from Patient to Health Care Personnel

	Bacteria	Viruses	Parasites
DIRECT	Group A Streptococci *Staphylococcus aureus* Syphilis	Herpes simplex Herpes zoster	Pediculosis Scabies
RESPIRATORY (aerosol and contact with infected respiratory secretions)	*Haemophilus influenzae* Meningococcus Pertussis Tuberculosis	Adenovirus Influenza Measles Mumps Parainfluenza Parvovirus B19 Respiratory syncytial virus Rhinovirus Rubella Varicella	
FECAL-ORAL	Campylobacter *Escherichia coli* Salmonella Shigella	Enteroviruses Hepatitis A, E Rotavirus	Cryptosporidium *Giardia lamblia*
BLOODBORNE (needlestick, mucosal spray, and nonintact skin contact with infected blood and body fluids)		Cytomegalovirus Hepatitis B, C Human immunodeficiency virus	

nal tract after being swallowed. Transmission by this fecal-oral route could be interrupted by removing the virus contaminating the individual's hands with a routine soap and water handwash. A second example is provided by transmission of respiratory viruses (e.g., rhinovirus, respiratory syncytial virus), which are excreted in nasal secretions and may be in droplets expelled during coughing. These viruses in droplets may be transferred to the well person by way of the air. Susceptible mucosal sites would be inoculated as the health care worker breathes the droplet-contaminated air. The frequency of transmission of agents through the air is probably small, although this is not known for certain. On the other hand, viruses in nasal secretions may contaminate the hands of the patient and articles in the environment. Transfer to the hands of the health care worker occurs during contact with contaminated articles or the hands and nasal secretions of the infected patient. Inoculation, the final step in transmission, requires that the hands of the health care worker contact the lining of the worker's nose or eye so as to deposit the virus on the mucosa. This self-inoculation step could be interrupted by washing the virus off of hands before mucosal contact, such as nose and/or eye rubbing.

What can be done to prevent transfer of infectious pathogens in the health care workplace? Constant cleaning of equipment, furniture, and common use items and surfaces (e.g., charts, counter tops, phone, doorknob) is an obvious means of reducing environmental contamination with skin contaminants, respiratory material, feces, and other blood and body fluids. The consistent use of barrier precautions and isolation techniques further interrupts transmission. All agree that handwashing is the control measure that is the most effective method of preventing self-inoculation of pathogens. The availability of handwash facilities and the importance of the repetitive use of these facilities by personnel cannot be overemphasized as the key to avoiding becoming infected in the health care workplace.

chapter 2

FUNDAMENTALS OF INFECTION PROTECTION

Frequent handwashing, the use of barrier garments and personal protective equipment, and contaminated waste management are the cornerstone of infection protection for the health care worker. The following techniques require a knowledge of the available equipment, its recommended use in different settings, and its incorporation into one's routine practice in the health care workplace.

HANDWASHING

Handwashing remains the single most effective means of removing organisms acquired from infected patients. Handwashing consists of a soap and water wash for longer than 10 seconds using a rubbing action that creates a lather over the entire hand surface and is then fully rinsed with running water. Hands should be dried with disposable or single-use towels or an air dryer.

BARRIER PRECAUTIONS

Gloves

Gloves reduce the incidence of hand contamination with infective material, which reduces the opportunity for personnel to become infected and/or the organisms to spread to other personnel and patients. Gloves, however, should never replace handwashing, which actually eliminates the pathogens. Hands should be washed whenever gloves are changed. Gloves should be changed between care of different patients and between care of different body parts on the same patient.

Gloves should be made of materials impervious to infectious agents for the entire period of time they are in use. They should be of sufficient quality so that the necessary sense of touch and technical skills of the health care worker are retained; they should be of sufficient strength to prevent tearing and perforation during use.

The number of organisms on a contaminated needle have been shown to decrease when punctured through a glove. The glove, therefore, may provide increased protection by reducing the pathogen inoculum during a needlestick injury.

Double gloving may increase protection in the high-risk setting.

Currently, available gloves should not be washed or used with petroleum-based hand creams. Detergents, antibacterial agents, and petroleum-based hand creams can increase the glove permeability and may actually cause leaking of infectious material through unrecognized breaks.

Gowns

Gowns should be worn when soiling of clothes or scrub suits with infective materials is likely. Gowns that are resistant or impervious to fluid should be used when soaking or large amounts of fluid splash or spill are likely. Surgical caps or hoods and/or leggings, shoe covers, or boots should be worn in instances when gross contamination is likely.

Masks

Masks protect the health care worker from small-particle droplet nuclei that travel for larger distances and from large-particle droplets that surround the patient for approximately 3 feet.

High-efficiency disposable masks are better than cotton or paper masks in filtering small-particle droplet nuclei. Masks should be changed when required for prolonged periods or if they become wet because they become less efficient filters over time.

A newer, better-fitting, high-efficiency mask called a disposable particulate respirator provides a tight face seal and is a better filter for droplet particle nuclei. These masks are currently recommended for health care personnel who share air space with patients who have tuberculosis.

Goggles, Eye Protection, and Face Shields

Masks in combination with goggles, glasses with disposable side shields, or face shields are suggested for any procedure where splashing or spraying of blood or other potentially infectious material onto nasal, oral, or eye mucosa is likely.

UNIVERSAL PRECAUTIONS

In 1985, primarily resulting from the AIDS epidemic and secondarily from the knowledge that hepatitis B infection is a significant work-related infection, medical recommendations and, subsequently, governmental regulations have evolved requiring very specific preventive guidelines to reduce the risk of transmission of bloodborne pathogens in the workplace.

In 1991, the Occupational Safety and Health Administration (OSHA) published specific requirements (Occupational Exposure to Bloodborne Pathogens; Final Rule. Federal Register, December 6, 1991) requiring employers to follow specific guidelines for employees who, as a result of their duties, could have skin, eye, mucous membrane, or parenteral contact with blood or other potentially infectious materials (OPIM). OPIM is the current terminology for body fluids, tissues, specimens, etc. that represent a possible infectious danger to the health care worker.

The following infection control practices should be learned, understood, and practiced religiously in the care of all patients. The specific guidelines for Universal Precautions include:

HEPATITIS B VACCINE

Hepatitis B vaccine must be provided free of charge for all nonimmune health care workers who have the reasonable anticipation of exposure to blood and other potentially infectious materials in the health care workplace. Employees may refuse vaccination but must sign an informed refusal, which is retained in their personal file.

Gloves are to be worn for touching:

- Blood;
- Any body fluid contaminated with blood;
- Amniotic fluid;
- Pericardial fluid;
- Peritoneal fluid;
- Pleural fluid;
- Synovial fluid;
- Cerebrospinal fluid;
- Saliva in dental procedures;

- Semen;
- Vaginal secretions;
- Mucous membranes;
- Patient skin that is abnormal or cut;
- Any surface or object soiled with blood or above body fluids;
- Any surface or object that could be contaminated with blood or other potentially infectious materials (e.g., outside of patient specimen container);
- Performing vascular access or invasive procedures.

Gloves should be changed when torn, between contact with different body parts on the same patient, and after contact with each patient. Gloves should be removed before touching clean items (e.g., phone, doorknob, chart). After removing gloves, hands should always be washed.

HANDWASHING

Handwashing should be:

- Immediate and thorough if contaminated with blood or other potentially infectious materials;
- Performed after each patient contact;
- Performed after glove removal.

NEEDLES, SHARP INSTRUMENTS, AND OTHER DEVICES

These should be handled with special care, which includes:

- Never recapping needles;
- Never bending or breaking needles;
- Never removing needles from disposable syringes;
- Immediate disposal after use of all disposable syringes and needles, scalpel blades, and other sharp instruments in a color-coded or labeled leak-proof puncture-resistant, closable needle box, or contaminated materials container (CMC);
- Immediate placement after use of reusable needles and sharp instruments in a labeled or color-coded, leak-proof puncture-resistant container for processing;

- Removing needle from a clean Vacutainer holder with a needle removal device, not the hands;
- Discarding Vacutainer holder and attached needle if visibly bloody;
- Never picking up broken glassware with one's hands; use mechanical means such as forceps or brush and dust pan.

GOWNS

Gowns are worn to prevent blood and other potentially infectious materials from having direct contact with personal clothing, skin, or mucous membranes. Recommendations for use include:

- Never using cloth lab coats, scrub suits, or street clothes as an effective barrier to blood or body fluids;
- The use of fluid-resistant gowns or plastic aprons if soiling of clothes with blood or other potentially infectious material is likely;
- The use of disposable fluid-resistant caps, sleeves, boots, and leggings if the potential for exposure is likely and added protection is warranted;
- The removal of personal protective equipment immediately upon leaving the worker area and placement of these items in a designated container;
- The immediate removal of a gown, scrub, etc. that is penetrated with blood or other potentially infectious materials in a way that does not contaminate the head or face; if this is not possible with a pullover item, it should be cut off with scissors.

MASKS, PROTECTIVE EYE WEAR, OR FACE SHIELDS

These are worn to prevent exposure of mucous membranes of the mouth, nose, and eyes during procedures that are likely to create droplets of blood or other body fluids. They are required:

- Whenever spraying, splashing, or splattering of face is possible;
- During all dental, surgical, laboratory, and postmortem procedures;
- During suctioning, intubation, bronchoscopy, endoscopy, and during the cleaning of these instruments.

Eyeglasses with solid side shields with a face mask provide minimal protection. Goggles with a face mask provide reasonable protection. Face shields provide maximum protection.

CARDIOPULMONARY MASKS, MOUTHPIECES, RESUSCITATION BAGS AND OTHER VENTILATION DEVICES

These should be:

- Used as the alternative to mouth-to-mouth resuscitation;
- Readily available in areas where the need for resuscitation is predictable.

DERMATITIS

Health care workers with exudate lesions or weeping dermatitis must:

- Avoid direct patient care and handling of patient care equipment until their skin condition resolves.

LINENS, PERSONAL CLOTHING, SCRUB SUITS

Items contaminated with blood and other potentially infectious material should be:

- Handled with gloves;
- Placed in fluid-proof bags;
- Laundered or disinfected on site, even if the articles are personal items.

ENVIRONMENTAL CLEANING

Blood or other potentially infectious material spills should be promptly removed and disinfected using:

- Gloves;
- Freshly made solution of one part bleach to nine parts water;
- Flooding spill with bleach solution for 10 minutes prior to cleaning;
- Paper towels.

Never pick up broken glassware with the hands. Do not eat, drink, apply cosmetics, or handle contact lenses in patient work areas.

EXPOSURE

Know what a significant blood or other potentially infectious material exposure is, what is not an exposure, and what to do if exposed.

Exposure to blood or other potentially infectious material *is* defined as:

- Injury with a contaminated sharp object (e.g., needlestick, scalpel cut);
- Spills or splashes of blood or other potentially infectious material onto nonintact skin (e.g., cuts, hangnails, dermatitis, abrasions, chapped skin) or onto a mucous membrane (e.g., mouth, nose, eye);
- Blood exposure covering a large area of normal skin.

An exposure does *not* occur from:

- Handling food trays or furniture;
- Pushing wheelchairs, stretchers;
- Using rest rooms or phones;
- Personal contact with patients (e.g., giving information, touching intact skin, bathing, giving a back rub, shaking hands);
- Doing clerical or administrative duties for a patient.

If hands or other skin surfaces are exposed to blood or other potentially infectious material:

- Wash the area with soap for at least 10 seconds;
- Rinse with running water for at least 10 seconds.

If your eyes, nose, or mouth are splashed with blood or body fluids:

- Irrigate affected area with large amounts of water.

If a skin cut, puncture, or lesion is exposed to blood or other potentially infectious material:

- Wash with soap and water for at least 10 seconds;
- Rinse with 70% isopropyl alcohol.

Report any exposure incident to Employee Health as soon as possible. Know who to contact, where to go, and what to do if inadvertently exposed. Every health care worker should know where to find the **EXPOSURE CONTROL PLAN** that is specific for his/her place of employment. Important resources are Employee Health, the Emergency Room, and Infection Control/Hospital Epidemiology. The most important recommendation in any accidental exposure is to seek advice and intervention immediately because efficacy of prophylaxis and/or treatment may depend on the exposure to treatment interval (e.g., HBIG after exposure to hepatitis B). Additionally, reporting a work-related exposure is required for subsequent medical care, worker's compensation, etc. documentation. Should an exposure incident not be reported, it is difficult to prove in retrospect that an illness was caused by a work-related rather than a personal exposure.

The following **CATEGORY-SPECIFIC ISOLATION GUIDELINES** should be, in concert with universal precautions, carefully utilized in the care of specific contagious illnesses and diseases known to be controlled by these precautions.

ISOLATION CATEGORIES

Strict Isolation

Strict isolation is the most restrictive category of isolation designed to prevent the transmission of highly virulent and contagious pathogens spread by both direct contact and airborne nuclei. Specific instructions for strict isolation include:

- Private room;
- Negative pressure ventilation;
- Masks at all times;
- Gowns at all times;
- Gloves at all times;
- Handwashing after glove removal.

Examples of patients with diseases requiring strict isolation include those with:

- Pharyngeal diphtheria;
- Varicella;
- Lassa fever and other viral hemorrhagic fevers.

Contact Isolation

Contact isolation is designed to prevent diseases transmitted by close and direct contact and not by airborne droplet nuclei. Specific instructions for contact isolation include:

- Private room;
- Masks when close to patient to prevent large-droplet transmission;
- Gowns if soiling likely;
- Gloves for touching infective material;
- Handwashing after glove removal.

Examples of patients with diseases requiring contact isolation include those with:

- Major staphylococcal infections;
- Major wound infections;
- Pediatric patients with respiratory infections (e.g., respiratory syncytial virus);
- Rubella;
- Scabies;
- Pediculoses.

Respiratory Isolation

Respiratory isolation is designed to prevent transmission of diseases spread by large airborne droplets. Specific instructions for respiratory isolation include:

- Private room;
- Mask when close to patient to prevent droplet transmission;
- Handwashing.

Examples of patients with diseases requiring respiratory isolation include those with:

- Mumps;
- Pertussis;
- Measles;
- Meningococcal disease;
- *Haemophilus influenzae* Type B disease.

Tuberculosis (AFB) Isolation

Tuberculosis isolation is to be used for all patients with known, suspected, or at high risk for having tuberculosis. Specific instructions for tuberculosis (AFB) isolation include:

- Private room;
- Negative pressure ventilation;
- Masks (better fitting, increased filtering, particulate respirators);
- Gown, if soiling likely;
- Handwashing.

Enteric Precautions

Enteric precautions are isolation guidelines designed to prevent infections transmitted by contact, direct and indirect, with feces. Specific instructions for enteric precautions include:

- Gowns, if soiling likely;
- Gloves for touching infective material;
- Handwashing after glove removal.

Examples of patients with diseases requiring enteric precautions include those with:

- Hepatitis A, E;
- Cholera;
- Salmonella;
- Shigella;
- Campylobacter;
- Giardia;
- Rotavirus.

Drainage/Secretion Precautions

Drainage secretion precautions are isolation guidelines designed to prevent transmission of infections by direct or indirect contact with secretions from an infected body site. Specific instructions for drainage/secretion precautions include:

- Gowns, if soiling likely;
- Gloves for touching infective material;
- Handwashing after glove removal.

Examples of patients with diseases requiring drainage/secretion precautions include those with:

- Conjunctivitis;
- Herpes simplex;
- Localized Herpes zoster;

- Papillomavirus;
- Syphilis.

Blood/Body Fluid Precautions

Blood and body fluid precautions is an older designation that antedated Universal Blood and Body Fluid Precautions and Universal Bloodborne Pathogen Precautions. Regardless of the title, the intent of the precaution is to prevent transmission of bloodborne pathogens by direct or indirect contact, inoculation with sharp instruments or needles, or mucosal spray with infected blood or other potentially infectious materials. Specific instructions are detailed fully under Universal Precautions and include:

- Fluid-resistant gowns, if soiling likely;
- Gloves for touching infective material;
- Mask in combination with glasses with side shields, goggles, or face shield, if spray likely;
- Care with needles and sharp instruments.

Examples of patients with diseases requiring blood/body fluid precautions include those with:

- Hepatitis B, C, D;
- Cytomegalovirus;
- Human Immunodeficiency Virus (HIV) infections and Acquired Immune Deficiency Syndrome (AIDS);
- Leptospirosis;
- Malaria.

chapter 3

EMPLOYEE HEALTH

The function of an effective infection control program for the health care worker requires an Employee Health Department that:

- Identifies health care workers at high risk of acquiring or developing severe infections with pathogens acquired at work;
- Educates health care workers on routine health maintenance, infection control techniques, and the expedient reporting of exposure to infectious pathogens;
- Requires and provides vaccine protection for all susceptible health care workers;
- Requires and administrates a user-friendly post exposure plan that includes prophylaxis if available, counseling, surveillance for the development of infection, and treatment as needed;
- Provides personal protective equipment and required laundering, if required, at no cost to the employee.

HIGH-RISK EMPLOYEE

All health care workers who have direct patient care responsibilities should protect themselves from infection by frequent handwashing, using available barrier protection (personal protective equipment), receiving available immunizations, and having a fundamental working and up-to-date knowledge of infection risks, transmission, and available protective equipment and procedure.

High-risk health care workers should additionally obtain information from their personal physicians and Employee Health regarding what limited, if any, infected patients they should avoid having direct patient responsibility for and what additional protective measures they should utilize.

The following comments on specific high-risk health care workers are general recommendations for the health care setting. It is important, however, to remember that these recommendations should be maintained in personal practices at home because the routine care of children (particularly those in day care and preschool) and older people in the household may pose greater risks of transmitting these same pathogens in a setting where scrupulous handwashing, environmental cleaning, and personal protective equipment are not the routine.

Health Care Worker with Chronic Cardiac Disease

The major risks for this group of patients are respiratory viral and bacterial infection that lead to lower respiratory tract infection and result in further cardiac decompensation. Some of the problem pathogens are:

- Adenovirus;
- Influenzae;
- Parainfluenzae;
- Pneumococcus;
- Respiratory syncytial virus.

Important preventive procedures are:

- Rigorous handwashing routines;
- Barrier protection;

- Yearly influenza vaccine;
- Increased vigilance during the winter months when these pathogens are prevalent and often unrecognized in hospitalized patients.

Health Care Worker with Chronic Pulmonary Disease (e.g., Cystic Fibrosis, Emphysema, Asthma)

The major risks for this group of health care workers are respiratory viral and bacterial infection that lead to worsening ventilatory status or exacerbate the underlying pulmonary disease. If the underlying disease is further being treated with immunosuppressive agents, this therapy then poses an additional risk of infection. Examples of the potential problem pathogens are:

- Adenovirus;
- Influenzae;
- Parainfluenzae;
- Pneumococcus;
- Respiratory syncytial virus;
- Tuberculosis.

    Important preventive procedures include:

- Rigorous handwashing routines;
- Barrier protection;
- Routine tuberculous screening;
- Yearly influenza vaccine;
- Increased vigilance during the winter months when these pathogens are prevalent and often unrecognized in hospitalized patients.

Health Care Worker with Chronic Skin Disease

Eczema is a common skin condition. Eczema, variants of eczema, and chronic dermatitis all increase the risk of hand colonization and subsequent infection with spread to the deeper layers of the skin, contiguous skin, or by self-inoculation to other sites. Problem pathogens for these patients are:

- Group A streptococcus;
- Herpes simplex virus;
- *Staphylococcus aureus.*

Careful treatment of the underlying skin condition to maintain skin health and integrity is probably the most effective preventive modality. Additional preventive procedures include:

- Careful handwashing with soaps that do not exacerbate underlying condition;
- Continued use of lotions that are known to be sterile;
- Gloving;
- Gown and disposable sleeve protection;
- Avoidance of all direct contact with all skin lesions and wounds.

Health Care Worker with Chronic Hemolytic Disease (e.g., Sickle Cell Disease)

There are a few very specific pathogens that cause severe disease in patients with sickle cell disease. These pathogens include:

- *Haemophilus influenzae;*
- *Mycoplasma pneumoniae*;
- Parvovirus B19;
- *Pneumococcus*;
- *Salmonella.*

Since most of these pathogens are certainly as common, if not more so, out of the health care setting, it is important for persons with chronic hemolytic disease to maintain the following preventive procedures in both their professional and personal environments:

- Careful handwashing;
- Careful environmental cleaning around children and adults with upper and lower respiratory infections;
- Gloving for handling all pediatric respiratory secretions.

Health Care Worker with an Indwelling Device (e.g., Vascular Catheter, Ventriculoperitoneal Shunt, Tenchoff Catheter)

From our understanding of device-associated infection, many of which are in immunocompromised patients, the infections usually result from infection with one's own skin or other flora.

Important pathogens as causes of device-related infection and specifically vascular devices are:

- Coagulase-negative staphylococci;
- *Staphylococcus aureus;*
- *Candida albicans.*

Important preventive procedures include:

- Vigilant aseptic care and maintenance of the device;
- The use of sterile gloves in touching or manipulation of the device because hand colonization of health care workers may include hospital-acquired hand flora;
- Careful maintenance of skin integrity around or over the device;
- Careful, complete covering of the device at all times in the workplace.

Health Care Worker with Infants at Home

Many health care workers with infants less than 1 year of age at home are concerned that they can bring pathogens home from the health care workplace and infect their susceptible children. An immune health care worker who is exposed to varicella, for example, is not going to become a silent "carrier" of this pathogen. However, pathogens to which the health care worker is not immune or that carry only partial or incomplete immunity may infect health care workers with a severe, mild, or asymptomatic infection that they can easily transmit to their family members. Examples of these pathogens are:

- Influenza;
- Pertussis;
- Respiratory syncytial virus;
- Rotavirus;
- Tuberculosis.

Important preventive procedures for health care workers with infants at home are:

- Yearly influenza vaccine;
- Routine tuberculosis screening;
- Prior immunity or vaccine for polio, measles, mumps, hepatitis B, rubella;
- Early medical evaluation for all infectious illnesses;
- Routine immunization of infants;
- Careful handwashing and removal of hospital attire before touching infant and infant environment;
- Early prophylaxis and/or therapy if exposed or infected;
- Avoid infant contact if infected.

Health Care Worker Who Is, Could Be, or Anticipates Being Pregnant

Pregnancy for the health care worker should not be viewed as an obstacle to continued work in the health care workplace. In fact, with universal precautions, the environmental cleaning and protective procedures required for appropriate patient care, the vigilant health care worker is, in my opinion, at far less risk than a preschool teacher, day care provider, or the mother of children with many playmates in the home.

Some of the pathogens of concern to the pregnant health care worker are:

- Cytomegalovirus;
- Hepatitis E;
- Influenza;
- Measles;
- Mumps;
- Parvovirus B19;
- Rubella;
- Tuberculosis;
- Varicella zoster virus.

Important preventive procedures include:

- Documented immunity or immunization prior to pregnancy for rubella, mumps, measles, polio, hepatitis B;
- Yearly influenza vaccine;
- Routine tuberculosis screening;
- Early medical evaluation for all infectious illnesses;
- Early prophylaxis and/or therapy if exposed or infected.

The pregnant worker should assume that all of her patients are potentially infected with cytomegalovirus and other "silent" pathogens and use gloves followed by careful handwashing when handling all body fluids, secretions, and excretions.

Health Care Worker Who is Immunocompromised (e.g., Cancer, Neutropenia, Transplant, HIV-Infected, Steroid Therapy, Immunosuppressive Agents)

Any immunocompromised health care worker may become infected from his/her own normal flora or from pathogens acquired in the home or work environment. It has been shown that the health care worker's "normal" skin, gastrointestinal, nasopharyngeal flora, etc. may change over time to include organisms more commonly found in the health care setting where he/she works. As a result, this new flora, which would be innocuous in the immunologically normal individual, may be pathogenic for the at-risk individual. It is important that the immunocompromised health care worker understands these risks, discuss them with his/her personal physician, make them known to Employee Health, and carefully maintain infection control practices at work and at home to reduce the risk of acquiring high-risk pathogens.

"Usual" organisms in the health care workplace that can cause infection in the immunocompromised individual include:

- *Candida* species;
- Coagulase-negative staphylococcus;
- *Staphylococcus aureus*;
- Enteric Gram-negative rods.

Other potential infectors that can be a cause of severe infection in the immunocompromised health care worker include:

- Adenovirus;
- Aspergillus;
- Cryptosporidia;
- Cytomegalovirus;
- Enterovirus;
- *Giardia lamblia*;
- Herpes simplex virus;
- Influenza;
- Measles;
- Microsporidia;
- *Mycoplasma pneumoniae*;
- Norwalk agent;
- Parainfluenzae;
- Parvovirus B19;
- *Pneumococcus*;
- *Pneumocystis carinii*;

- Poliovirus;
- Respiratory syncytial virus;
- Rotavirus;
- *Salmonella*;
- Tuberculosis;
- Varicella zoster virus;
- *Vibrio*;
- *Yersinia*.

Regardless of the reservoir, both sources of organisms need to be avoided. Important protective procedures for the immunocompromised health care worker include:

- Knowledge of immune status to rubella, mumps, measles, polio, hepatitis B, and appropriate immunization;
- Yearly influenzae vaccine;
- Routine tuberculosis screening;
- Early medical evaluation for all infectious illnesses;
- Early prophylaxis and/or therapy if exposed or infected;
- The assumption that all patients are potentially infected or colonized with potential pathogens and the routine use of gloves followed by careful handwashing when handling all body fluids, tissues, secretions, and excretions;
- The preference, if staffing can be arranged, to care for patients with no known infectious illnesses.

EMPLOYEE EDUCATION

The Employee Health Department should be an educational resource for information on infectious pathogens in the health care workplace. This department, in concert with the infection control service, should provide annual training for all employees on:

- Routine health maintenance;
- Available vaccines;
- Universal precautions and isolation categories;
- Exposure plans.

With new pathogens being isolated, new diseases and their transmission described, and new prophylactic regimens and treatment available, it is mandatory that personnel have an up-to-date working knowledge of infection control and know where and what the available services, equipment, and therapies are for the health care worker.

IMMUNIZATION RECOMMENDATIONS

All employees should be screened by history and/or serologic testing to document their immune status to:

- Diphtheria/Tetanus;
- Hepatitis B;
- Mumps;
- Polio;
- Rubella;
- Rubeola;
- Varicella.

Vaccine protection should be provided for all employees who are nonimmune and who do not have contraindications to receiving the vaccine. The following vaccines are routinely recommended for health care workers with patient contact:

- Diphtheria/Tetanus;
- Hepatitis B (required by OSHA);
- Influenza;
- Mumps;
- Polio;
- Rubella;
- Rubeola;
- (Varicella—when available).

Tuberculosis screening and/or assessment should be a regular and routine responsibility of the Employee Health program.

EXPOSURE PLAN

Table 3.1 (page 30) outlines the pathogens and exposures that employees may encounter that require Employee Health notification, counsel, prophylaxis if available and indicated, and ongoing surveillance for infection and treatment if infected.

Table 3.1.
Exposure Plan

Infectious Pathogen	Postexposure Prophylaxis for Susceptible Health Care Workers	Treatment of Infected Health Care Workers
Conjunctivitis, viral		
Cytomegalovirus		
Group A streptococcus		X
Haemophilus influenzae Type B	Rifampin	X
Hepatitis A	Immune globulin	
Hepatitis B	Hepatitis B immune globulin Hepatitis B vaccine	
Hepatitis C	Immune Globulin	
Herpes simplex virus		X
Human Immunodeficiency Virus and Acquired Immunodeficiency Syndrome	Azidothymidine*	
Influenza A	Amantadine	X
Measles	Immune globulin Measles vaccine	

*Experimental.

Table 3.1.—*continued*
Exposure Plan

Infectious Pathogen	Postexposure Prophylaxis for Susceptible Health Care Workers	Treatment of Infected Health Care Workers
Meningococcus	Rifampin	X
Mumps		
Parvovirus B19		
Pediculosis		X
Pertussis	Erythromycin	X
Rabies	Human rabies immune globulin Rabies vaccine	
Rubella	Immune globulin	
Salmonella		X
Scabies		X
Shigella		X
Staphylococcus aureus		X
Syphilis		X
Tuberculosis		X
Varicella/Disseminated herpes zoster	Varicella zoster immune globulin	X
Contaminated needlestick or sharp injury	X	
Mucosal or nonintact skin exposure to blood and body fluids	X	

chapter 4

DISEASE-SPECIFIC PRECAUTIONS

This chapter is designed to be a ready reference for infection control measures to be instituted when caring for a patient whose illness (e.g., bloodstream infection, conjunctivitis, gastroenteritis) is known but the specific infectious pathogen has not yet been identified. Specific guidelines are provided on:

- What patient materials are infectious;
- How these infectious materials are transmitted;
- The recommended patient isolation category (Table 4.1, p. 34).

Once the infecting pathogen is known, specific precautions for that organism can be instituted per the guidelines in Chapter 5.

ISOLATION CATEGORIES

Strict Isolation

- Private room;
- Negative pressure ventilation;
- Masks at all times;

- Gowns at all times;
- Gloves at all times;
- Handwashing after glove removal.

Contact Isolation

- Private room;
- Masks when close to patient;
- Gowns, if soiling likely;
- Gloves for touching infective material;
- Handwashing after glove removal.

Respiratory Isolation

- Private room;
- Mask when close to patient;
- Handwashing.

Tuberculosis (AFB) Isolation

- Private room;
- Negative pressure ventilation;
- Masks (better fitting, increased filtering, particulate respirators);
- Gown, if soiling likely;
- Handwashing.

Enteric Precautions

- Gowns, if soiling likely;
- Gloves for touching infective material;
- Handwashing after glove removal.

Drainage/Secretion Precautions

- Gowns, if soiling likely;
- Gloves for touching infective material;
- Handwashing after glove removal.

Blood/Body Fluid Precautions

- Fluid-resistant gowns if soiling likely;
- Gloves for touching infective material;
- Mask in combination with glasses with side shields, goggles, or face shield, if spray likely;
- Care with needles and sharp instruments.

Table 4.1.
Recommended Patient Isolation Categories

Disease	Infected Material	Method of Transmission in the Health Care Workplace	Recommended Isolation/ Precaution
Bloodstream infection (bacteremia, viremia, parasitemia)	Blood/body fluid Respiratory secretions	Needlestick/sharp injury Hand to eye/nose Aerosol Mucous membrane or intact skin contact or splash	Blood/body fluid Contact Strict
Common cold	Respiratory secretions Fomites	Hand to eye/nose	Contact
Conjunctivitis	Purulent eye drainage Fomites	Hand to eye/nose	Contact
Gastroenteritis/diarrhea	Feces Fomites	Hand to mouth	Enteric
Gingivostomatitis	Respiratory secretions Fomites	Hand to mucous membrane/skin	Contact
Hepatitis	Blood and body fluids Feces	Needlestick/sharp injury Hand to mouth Mucous membrane or non-intact skin contact or splash	Blood/body fluid Enteric

Table 4.1.—*continued*
Recommended Patient Isolation Categories

Disease	Infected Material	Method of Transmission in the Health Care Workplace	Recommended Isolation/ Precaution
Meningitis	Respiratory secretions Feces Fomites	Hand to eye/nose Hand to mouth	Contact Enteric
Pediculosis (lice)	Infested skin Fomites	Direct contact	Contact (no mask)
Pneumonia	Respiratory secretions	Hand to eye/nose Aerosol	Contact Tuber- culosis
Skin/wound infections	Lesions Purulent exudate Fomites	Hand to skin Direct contact	Drainage/se- cretion

chapter 5

PATHOGEN-SPECIFIC PRECAUTIONS

This section is designed to be a ready reference for pathogen-specific infection control.

Each pathogen-specific infection has instructions for:

- What patient materials are infectious;
- The recommended isolation category for the infected patient;
- The availability of a protective vaccine;
- Recommended prophylaxis for an inadvertent exposure;
- Identification of health care workers at high risk of infection and/or severe infection.

ISOLATION CATEGORIES

Strict Isolation

- Private room;
- Negative pressure ventilation;
- Masks at all times;
- Gowns at all times;

- Gloves at all times;
- Handwashing after glove removal.

Contact Isolation

- Private room;
- Masks when close to patient;
- Gowns, if soiling likely;
- Gloves for touching infective material;
- Handwashing after glove removal.

Respiratory Isolation

- Private room;
- Mask when close to patient;
- Handwashing.

Tuberculosis (AFB) Isolation

- Private room;
- Negative pressure ventilation;
- Masks (better fitting, increased filtering, particulate respirators);
- Gown, if soiling likely;
- Handwashing.

Enteric Precautions

- Gowns, if soiling likely;
- Gloves for touching infective material;
- Handwashing after glove removal.

Drainage/Secretion Precautions

- Gowns, if soiling likely;
- Gloves for touching infective material;
- Handwashing after glove removal.

Blood/Body Fluid Precautions

- Fluid-resistant gowns, if soiling likely;
- Gloves for touching infective material;
- Mask in combination with glasses with side shields, goggles, or face shield, if spray likely;
- Care with needles and sharp instruments.

Table 5.1
Pathogen-Specific Precautions

Infectious Disease	Infective Patient Material	Recommended Patient Isolation	Vaccine Prevention	Prophylaxis for Exposure	High-Risk Health Care Worker
Actinomycosis					
Adenovirus infection Respiratory	Respiratory secretions	Contact			• Chronic cardiac disease • Chronic pulmonary disease • Immunocompromised
Conjunctivitis	Purulent exudate	Drainage/secretion	*		
Gastroenteritis	Feces	Enteric			
Amebiasis	Feces	Enteric			
Anthrax	Lesion secretions	Drainage/secretion	*		
Arbovirus infection	Blood	Blood/body fluid	*		
Ascariasis					
Aspergillosis					• Immunocompromised
Astrovirus infection	Feces	Enteric			

Babesiosis	Blood	Blood/body fluid
Bacillus cereus infection Skin infection	Purulent exudate	Drainage/secretion
Bacteroides infection Skin infection	Purulent exudate	Drainage/secretion
Balantidium coli infection		
Blastocystis hominis infection		
Blastomycosis		
Borrelia (relapsing fever)	Blood	Blood/body fluids Contact without mask until louse infestation is treated

* The available vaccines are not universally recommended for health care workers.

Table 5.1—*continued*
Pathogen-Specific Precautions

Infectious Disease	Infective Patient Material	Recommended Patient Isolation	Vaccine Prevention	Prophylaxis for Exposure	High-Risk Health Care Worker
Botulism					
Brucellosis Undulant fever					
Draining lesions	Purulent exudate	Contact			
Campylobacter infection	Feces	Enteric			• Immunocompromised
Candidiasis					• Indwelling device
Cat scratch disease					
Chlamydia infection Conjunctivitis	Purulent exudate	Drainage/ secretion			
Genital	Genital secretions	Drainage/ secretion			
Respiratory	Respiratory secretions	Contact			

Disease			
Cholera	Feces	Enteric	*
Clostridium difficile infection	Feces	Enteric	
Clostridial myonecrosis (gas gangrene)	Purulent exudate	Drainage/secretion	
Coccidiomycosis			
Coronavirus infection	Respiratory secretions	Contact	
Cryptococcus neoformans infection			
Cryptosporidiosis	Feces	Enteric	• Immunocompromised
Cutaneous larva migrans			
Cysticercosis			
Cytomegalovirus infection	Urine Respiratory secretions Blood	Blood/body fluid	• Immunocompromised • Pregnant

* The available vaccines are not universally recommended for health care workers.

Table 5.1—*continued*
Pathogen-Specific Precautions

Infectious Disease	Infective Patient Material	Recommended Patient Isolation	Vaccine Prevention	Prophylaxis for Exposure	High-Risk Health Care Worker
Diphtheria Cutaneous	Lesion secretions	Contact	Recommended	Booster dose of toxoid	
Pharyngeal	Respiratory secretions	Strict		Erythromycin or penicillin	
Ehrlichiosis	Blood	Blood/body fluid			
Enterovirus infection	Feces Respiratory secretions	Enteric			• Immunocompromised
Escherichia coli diarrhea	Feces	Enteric			
Filariasis					
Giardiasis	Feces	Enteric			• Chronic gastrointestinal disease • Immunocompromised

Gonococcal infection Genital	Genital secretions	Drainage/secretion			
Ophthalmia	Purulent exudate	Contact			
Granuloma inguinale	Infected secretions	Drainage/secretion			
Helicobacter pylori infection					• Sickle cell disease
Haemophilus influenzae infection	Respiratory secretions	Respiratory	*		
Hemorrhagic fevers Arenaviruses	Blood/body fluid	Strict		Ribavirin	
Bunyaviruses	Blood/body fluid	Strict		Ribavirin	
Hepatitis A	Feces	Enteric	Experimental	Immune globulin	

* The available vaccines are not universally recommended for health care workers.

Table 5.1—continued
Pathogen-Specific Precautions

Infectious Disease	Infective Patient Material	Recommended Patient Isolation	Vaccine Prevention	Prophylaxis for Exposure	High-Risk Health Care Worker
Hepatitis B	Blood/body fluid	Blood/body fluid	Recom-mended	Hepatitis B immune globulin Hepatitis B vaccine	
Hepatitis C	Blood/body fluid	Blood/body fluid		Immune globulin	
Hepatitis Delta virus	Blood/body fluid	Blood/body fluid			• HBsAg positive
Hepatitis E	Feces	Enteric			• Pregnant
Herpes simplex infection Disseminated	Lesion secretions Respiratory secretions	Contact			• Chronic skin disease • Immunocom-promised
Mucocutaneous (oral, skin, genital)	Lesion secretions	Drainage/ secretion			
Central nervous system					

	Lesion secretions	Drainage/secretion	Experimental	Varicella zoster immune globulin	Susceptible • Adults • Immunocompromised • Pregnant
Herpes zoster (shingles) Localized	Lesion secretions				
Disseminated	Lesion secretions Respiratory secretions	Strict (no mask for immune HCWs)	Experimental	Varicella zoster immune globulin	• Adults • Immunocompromised • Pregnant
Histoplasmosis					
Human immunodeficiency virus (HIV) infection and acquired immune deficiency syndrome (AIDS)	Blood/body fluid	Blood/body fluid		Azidothymidine (experimental)	
Hookworm					
Infectious mononucleosis	Respiratory secretions	Respiratory			

* The available vaccines are not universally recommended for health care workers.

Table 5.1—*continued*
Pathogen-Specific Precautions

Infectious Disease	Infective Patient Material	Recommended Patient Isolation	Vaccine Prevention	Prophylaxis for Exposure	High-Risk Health Care Worker
Influenza Adults	Respiratory secretions	Respiratory	Recom-mended	Amanta-dine	• Chronic car-diac disease • Chronic pulmonary disease • Immunocom-promised • Infants at home • Pregnant
Infants/young children	Respiratory secretions	Contact			
Isosporiasis	Feces	Enteric			
Jakob-Creutzfeldt disease	Blood Brain Spinal fluid	Blood/body fluid			
Kawasaki disease					
Legionellosis	Respiratory secretions				
Leishmaniasis					

			Recommended	Immune globulin Vaccine	
Leprosy					
Leptospirosis	Blood Urine	Blood/body fluid, gloves for handling urine			
Listeria monocytogenes infection	Genital secretions				
Lyme disease					
Lymphocytic choriomeningitis					
Lymphogranuloma venereum	Lesion secretions	Drainage/secretion			
Malaria	Blood	Blood/body fluid			
Malassezia furfur infection					
Measles	Respiratory secretions	Respiratory	Recommended	Immune globulin Vaccine	• Immunocompromised • Pregnant

*The available vaccines are not universally recommended for health care workers.

Table 5.1—continued
Pathogen-Specific Precautions

Infectious Disease	Infective Patient Material	Recommended Patient Isolation	Vaccine Prevention	Prophylaxis for Exposure	High-Risk Health Care Worker
Meningococcal infection	Respiratory secretions	Respiratory	*	Rifampin	
Microsporidiosis	Feces	Enteric			• Immunocom- promised
Molluscum contagiosum	Infected lesions	Drainage/ secretion			
Moraxella catarrhalis infection	Respiratory secretions				
Mumps	Respiratory secretions	Respiratory	Recom- mended		• Pregnant
Mycoplasma pneumoniae infection	Respiratory	Respiratory			• Immunocom- promised • Sickle cell disease
Nocardiosis					
Norwalk agent Gastroenteritis (calcivirus)	Feces	Enteric			• Immunocom- promised

Onchocerciasis			
Papillomavirus infection	Infected skin	Drainage/ secretion	
Paracoccidioid-omycosis			
Paragonimiasis			
Parainfluenza virus infection	Respiratory secretions	Contact	• Chronic cardiac disease • Chronic pulmonary disease • Immunocompromised
Parvovirus B19 infection Fifth disease			• Chronic hemolytic anemia • Immunocompromised • Pregnant
Aplastic crisis Chronic anemia Infected infants	Respiratory secretions Blood	Contact	
Pasteurella multocida infection	Purulent exudate	Drainage/ secretion	

* The available vaccines are not universally recommended for health care workers.

Table 5.1—*continued*
Pathogen-Specific Precautions

Infectious Disease	Infective Patient Material	Recommended Patient Isolation	Vaccine Prevention	Prophylaxis for Exposure	High-Risk Health Care Worker
Pediculosis (lice)	Infested skin	Contact without mask		Pediculicide if infested	
Pertussis	Respiratory secretions	Respiratory		Erythromycin	• Infants at home
Pinworm infection	Feces				
Plague Bubonic	Purulent exudate	Drainage/ secretion	*	Tetracycline or sulfonamide	
Pneumonic	Respiratory secretions	Strict			
Pneumococcal infection	Respiratory secretions		*		• Chronic cardiac disease • Chronic pulmonary disease • Immunocompromised • Sickle cell disease

			Recommended	Booster	
Pneumocystis carinii infection	Respiratory secretions				• Immunocompromised
Poliovirus infection	Feces Respiratory secretions	Enteric		Booster dose of vaccine	• Immunocompromised
Psittacosis	Respiratory secretions				
Q fever					
Rabies	Saliva Brain tissue Cerebrospinal fluid	Strict	*	Vaccine rabies immune globulin	
Rat-bite fever	Infected blood	Blood/body fluid			
Respiratory syncytial virus infection	Respiratory secretions	Contact			• Chronic/cardiac disease • Chronic pulmonary disease • Immunocompromised • Infants at home

* The available vaccines are not universally recommended for health care workers.

Table 5.1—*continued*
Pathogen-Specific Precautions

Infectious Disease	Infective Patient Material	Recommended Patient Isolation	Vaccine Prevention	Prophylaxis for Exposure	High-Risk Health Care Worker
Rickettsialpox					
Rocky Mountain spotted fever	Blood				
Roseola (HHV-6, exanthem subitum)	Respiratory secretions				
Rotavirus infection	Feces	Enteric	Experimental		• Immunocompromised • Infants at home
Rubella German measles	Respiratory secretions	Contact	Recommended	Immune globulin	• Pregnant
Congenital	Urine Respiratory secretions	Contact for first year of life			
Salmonellosis	Feces	Enteric	*		• Immunocompromised • Sickle cell disease

Scabies	Infested skin	Contact (no mask)	Scabicide if infested	
Schistosomiasis				
Shigellosis	Feces	Enteric		
Smallpox	Skin lesions Respiratory secretions	Strict	*	
Staphylococcal infection Skin	Infected skin Purulent exudate	Contact		• Chronic skin disease • Immunocompromised • Indwelling device
Pneumonia Lung abscess	Respiratory secretions	Contact		
Food poisoning				
Enterocolitis	Feces	Enteric		
Toxic shock syndrome	Genital secretions	Drainage/secretion		

* The available vaccines are not universally recommended for health care workers.

Table 5.1—*continued*
Pathogen-Specific Precautions

Infectious Disease	Infective Patient Material	Recommended Patient Isolation	Vaccine Prevention	Prophylaxis for Exposure	High-Risk Health Care Worker
Streptococcal infection, Group A Skin	Infected skin Purulent exudate	Contact			• Chronic skin disease • Rheumatic fever history
Pharyngitis	Respiratory secretions	Drainage/ secretion			
Pneumonia	Respiratory secretions	Contact			
Strongyloidiasis					
Syphilis	Lesion secretions Blood Cerebrospinal fluid	Drainage/ secretion Blood			
Tapeworm	Feces	Enteric			
Tetanus			Recommended		

Tinea infection	Lesion	Drainage/secretion		
Toxocariasis				
Toxoplasmosis	Blood			
Trichinosis				
Trichomoniasis	Genital secretions	Drainage/secretion		
Trichuriasis				
Trypanosomiasis	Blood Infected lesion	Blood/body fluid		
Tuberculosis Extrapulmonary	Exudate	Drainage/secretion	(Isoniazid if PPD becomes positive)	
Pulmonary	Respiratory secretions Airborne droplet nuclei	Tuberculosis	(Isoniazid if PPD becomes positive)	• Chronic pulmonary disease • Immunocompromised • Infants at home • Poorly controlled diabetes • Pregnant

* The available vaccines are not universally recommended for health care workers.

Table 5.1—continued
Pathogen-Specific Precautions

Infectious Disease	Infective Patient Material	Recommended Patient Isolation	Vaccine Prevention	Prophylaxis for Exposure	High-Risk Health Care Worker
Tularemia Draining lesion	Purulent exudate	Drainage/secretion			
Pulmonary	Respiratory secretions	Respiratory			
Typhus (epidemic)	Blood Lice	Contact without mask until pediculicide has been used	*		
Varicella (Chickenpox)	Respiratory secretions Lesion secretions	Strict (no mask for immune HCWs)	Experimental	Varicella zoster immune globulin	Susceptible • Adults • Immunocompromised • Pregnant

Vibrio infection			
Diarrhea (cholera)	Feces	Enteric	*
			• Immunocompromised
			• Liver disease
			• Low gastric acidity
Wounds	Infected lesions	Drainage/secretion	
Yersinia infection			
Enterocolitis	Feces	Enteric	• Immunocompromised

* The available vaccines are not universally recommended for health care workers.

INDEX

Page numbers followed by "t" denote tables.